Breathe Out

*Living Life to the Fullest, with
Emphysema, COPD, or Smoker's Lung*

Mary Callahan, RN

authorHOUSE®

AuthorHouse™
1663 Liberty Drive, Suite 200
Bloomington, IN 47403
www.authorhouse.com
Phone: 1-800-839-8640

First published by AuthorHouse 11/15/2007

ISBN: 978-1-4343-4855-5 (sc)

Library of Congress Control Number: 2007908840

Printed in the United States of America
Bloomington, Indiana

This book is printed on acid-free paper.

ACKNOWLEDGEMENTS

I want to thank Deb Brown for encouraging me to write the book, Renee Randazzo for all of her assistance, and Laura Howe for her illustrations.

Contents

Prologue ix

Chapter 1 1
Normal Lungs

Chapter 2 8
Basic Breathing Exercise, Parts 1 and 2

Chapter 3 13
When Good Lungs Go Bad

Chapter 4 32
Step 3—Breathing with the Diaphragm

Chapter 5 39
Complications of COPD

Chapter 6 54
Improving Your Exercise Tolerance

Chapter 7 60
Medications and Gadgets

Chapter 8 81
Activities of Daily Living

Chapter 9 87
Emotional Aspects Of COPD

Chapter 10 96
Stopping The Anxiety Cycle

Chapter 11 98
Medical tests and Lung Disease

Chapter 12 106
Make Your Diaphragm Work Harder

Chapter 13 107
    Nutrition and COPD

Chapter 14 113
    Things to Do in Bed with COPD

Chapter 15 117
    Review

Prologue

If your doctor has recently given you a diagnosis of chronic obstructive pulmonary disease (COPD) or emphysema, he probably explained the diagnosis and gave you some written information. You may have been referred to a pulmonary rehabilitation program. Both are worthwhile. But for many, the written information, usually a pamphlet provided by a drug company or the American Lung Association, is not enough. The same people may find that a pulmonary rehabilitation program is too much. It is time consuming, as much as three afternoons a week for twelve weeks. It s expensive, and insurance won't pay even part of the bill unless the disease is advanced enough.

This is a third alternative.

There is too much important information to be contained in a pamphlet. You deserve to learn how to minimize symptoms, even if at the time of diagnosis the symptoms are mild.

You need to learn how to avoid complications. It is those complications that can cause the disease to worsen and the symptoms to become severe.

It also helps to learn how to build your exercise tolerance and to keep it at the highest level possible. pulmonary rehabilitation programs are made for this. They put you on exercise equipment, monitoring your body's response as you improve.

Attending one of these programs is a great idea but not a necessity. You can accomplish the same thing on your own.

If you picked up this book because your doctor said you have "smoker's lung," you probably know in your heart that there is no such disease. Some doctors hesitate to label your condition as emphysema or COPD because they think they have nothing to offer you. Your doctor may think you don't need the black cloud of a diagnosis hanging over your head any longer than necessary.

With this book, and at least one new medication, your doctor now has something to offer.

That being said, if you have symptoms of shortness of breath or chronic cough, and have *diagnosed yourself* with "smoker's lung," you should get an official diagnosis. There are other conditions that cause the same symptoms. Why waste your time learning how to live with lung problems when you really have heart problems, for example? Plus, you may be delaying treatment for those other problems.

Since the subject of smoking has come up, of course you should quit. I doubt this is new information. But you don't have to be a nonsmoker to use this book. You have just as much right to health information as anyone else. Sometimes people who know they have caused their own illness by smoking feel so guilty about it that they don't think they deserve help. You do.

You might want to know that you are not alone. Smoking is not the only bad habit out there, and lung trouble is not the only result. At any given time, more than half the patients in the hospital are there because of their own bad habits or bad decisions. Some people overeat and end up with diabetes. Some drive recklessly and have car accidents. I don't know too many perfect people, so if you are not perfect either, read on anyway.

Now, you might be wondering how I got the privilege of telling people how to live with lung disease. I learned a little bit about lung disease in nursing school, thirty-six years ago. I learned more in respiratory therapy school two years later. But I mostly learned from the patients I taught for twenty years in New Mexico and another five in Maine.

The Lung Association of New Mexico hired me to teach a series of classes I called The Respiratory Disease Self-Care

Classes. We had them in the afternoons and evenings. We had them in Albuquerque and all over the state, even on American Indian reservations. Once I moved to Maine, I taught in two different pulmonary rehabilitation programs.

In the years I taught these classes, patients really taught me what they needed. It was very simple. The information the patients came back and thanked me for got a bigger place in the program. The parts no one ever thanked me for, or perhaps yawned while I taught, shrank and sometimes disappeared. This book contains the material that remained from those classes.

This book is not meant to educate doctors, nurses, or even respiratory therapists on lung disease. Reading it before a test might even make them flunk that test. The information is meant to be accessible to patients and make their conditions easier to understand. For example, COPD patients with an aspect of inflammation and swelling to their disease are no longer said to have an "asthmatic" component to their disease, but a "bronchospastic" component. The third disease under the heading COPD is now called bronchospastic disease, not asthma, in professional circles. The term *asthma* is reserved for the purer form of the disease, not complicated by emphysema and chronic bronchitis. But I have yet to have a patient tell me they have bronchospastic disease. They all still call it asthma, so I will call it asthma.

The classes I taught had two parts. The first half was lecture. The second half was practice of an exercise or a breathing technique. The book is set up the same way. Every other chapter is a lesson, starting with "Normal Lungs." The chapters in between give you something to do, an exercise or a breathing technique.

Enjoy.

Chapter 1

Normal Lungs

Something to think about

As organs of the body go, the lungs are fairly simple. They have only one job, and that is gas exchange: in with the good air, out with the bad; in with the oxygen, out with the carbon dioxide. Oxygen is what every organ and tissue of the body needs to stay alive. Carbon dioxide is the waste product of breathing. If you are wondering what a waste product is, think about the other things the body needs to stay alive:, food and water. They have waste products too.

The lungs have two major structures you need to know about, the air sacs and the bronchial tubes. The air sacs are where the gas exchange happens. The bronchial tubes deliver the air to the air sacs.

The interesting thing about the air sacs, also called alveoli, is that they are so small. In normal, healthy lungs there are 300 million of them, and they can be seen as individual sacs only under a microscope. Each one has tiny blood vessels, called capillaries, surrounding it that pick up the oxygen and drop off the carbon dioxide.

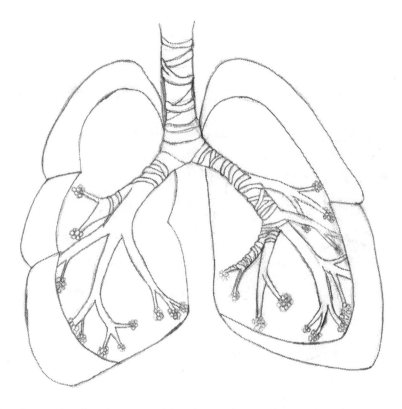

The bronchial tubes are like branches of a tree. They start with one big one, the trachea (or windpipe), and quickly start dividing and dividing and dividing again until there are thousands of them and they are very small as well. But the bronchial tubes are not just like garden hoses. They do more than deliver the goods. They also treat the air on its way to the air sacs.

The air sacs of the lungs, being small, are fairly fragile. They have to be kept warm, moist, and clean. The air we breathe is not always warm or moist enough. It is never clean enough. The lining of the bronchial tubes as well as the cavities behind the nose work to warm the air as it goes by and add humidity.

That is the easy part. The tricky part is filtering the dirt, pollution, and germs out of the air before it gets to the air sacs. As you can imagine, germs in the air sacs means infection, and that infection is called pneumonia. The bronchial tubes are called the defense mechanism of the lungs because they keep germs out of the air sacs and prevent pneumonia.

They do that because they have a very special lining. The lining produces a blanket of mucus that catches anything it touches like flypaper catches flies. As useful as it is to catch the germs before they can get to the air sacs, it is not good enough. The bronchial tubes also have to transport the germs out of the lungs.

They are able to move the mucus with the germs attached out of the lungs because of hairlike projections called cilia under the mucus blanket. They move like a field of wheat in the breeze, always beating upward. You may cough the bits of mucus out, but most of the time you swallow it without even knowing. It is normal and natural, and we all do it every day.

I have just described how healthy lungs work, but there is a little bit more to the respiratory system. To start with there is the mouth and nose. They are a part of the system because the air passes through them on the way to the lungs. The nose is part of the warming, humidifying, and filtering system. There are structures behind the nose: sinuses, nose hairs, and these curly bits of cartilage called turbinates that increase the surface area touched by the air on the way down. All that surface area begins the processes that are continued by the bronchial lining.

If you are a mouth breather, there is obviously less surface area for the air to touch on the way down, but there is still enough. The only real problem with breathing through your mouth is that you get a dry mouth out of it.

After the air goes through the nose or mouth, it heads toward the windpipe, also called the trachea. At a certain point there is a fork in the road, so to speak. There is a choice of going down the windpipe to the lungs or going down the esophagus toward the stomach. The air usually makes the right choice because there is a vacuum pulling the air into the lungs.

Food, drink, and saliva, meant to make the other choice, to go down the esophagus into the stomach, are more likely to make a mistake than air is. The vast majority of the time, they go the right way because a tiny flap called the epiglottis closes over the top of the windpipe every time you swallow, blocking entrance to the lungs. But from time to time, the epiglottis doesn't move fast enough and we get something "down the wrong pipe." For people with normal, healthy lungs this is an embarrassment, at worst. You cough and choke for a minute, and everyone jokes about doing a Heimlich maneuver on you.

If you already have breathing trouble, this coughing spell can be frightening. You may need a few minutes to recover when it is over, but it will be over. It is still just a little something "going down the wrong pipe."

The only thing you need to know about the windpipe is that it gets a little bigger around when you breathe in and a little smaller around when you breathe out. This is important because all the rest of the tubes leading into the lungs do the same, all the way down to the tiniest ones. Remember that when we talk about diseases of the lungs.

Another crucial part of the respiratory system are the muscles of breathing. Understanding how they work will help a great deal with symptom control.

The major muscle of breathing is the diaphragm. It is a large dome-shaped muscle that separates the chest cavity from the abdominal cavity. It sits high and rounded when you are resting between breaths. When the brain signals that you need another breath in, the diaphragm pulls down, lower and flatter, increasing the size of the chest cavity and creating a vacuum filled by the incoming air.

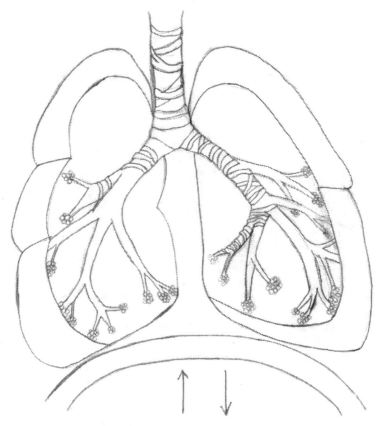

Breathing out is just the diaphragm moving back into its resting position.

In normal resting breathing, the diaphragm does almost all of the work. Other muscles that help a little are in the upper chest, between the ribs. When you are really working hard to breathe, like running a marathon, you might call on muscles in the neck and shoulders as well. All those muscles of breathing that ARE NOT the diaphragm are called the accessory muscles of respiration. They are extra help, there when you need them.

Lastly, when it comes to breathing, the brain plays a role. It tells you when to take each breath and how deep a breath it should be. This all goes back to what the job of the lungs really is: gas exchange. The brain controls your breathing so you exchange just the right amount of the gases, oxygen and carbon dioxide. You don't have to think about it. It all happens automatically.

The most important thing to remember about the role of the brain in breathing is that the brain will never scream, "Breathe out! Breathe out!" If you are short of breath, your brain will be screaming, "Breathe in. I need more oxygen," even if that is not what you really need.

Chapter 2

Basic Breathing Exercise, Parts 1 and 2

Something to Do

This chapter contains the most important information in the book. Seriously. If you learn nothing else but how to control your shortness of breath with breathing techniques, then you have still learned enough to change your life.

I call the exercise the "basic" breathing exercise because it is the heart of so many other things you will learn. When you learn how to improve your exercise tolerance, this exercise will be basic to it. When you learn how to control stress, this exercise will be crucial to it. When you learn how to carry groceries in the house without shortness of breath, guess what? This exercise is how you'll do it.

It is a three-step exercise. The first two steps are easy. If you don't already know them, you will learn them quickly. In spite of that, I recommend that you practice just those two steps for a few days before you add the last step. You may have used the technique to rescue yourself from shortness of breath, but you probably haven't used it to *prevent* shortness of breath. With practice you can learn to use the technique in a calm, controlled manner any time you see trouble coming.

Here goes:

Step 1—Pursed-lip breathing

Pursed-lip breathing means breathing out against lips that are partly closed, creating a back pressure felt all the way down into your lungs. It helps because that back pressure holds bronchial tubes open so you can exhale completely. You will learn that in COPD breathing tubes have a tendency to collapse, trapping air behind them and making it difficult to get the next breath in. Sometimes mucus plugs play a role in the air being trapped. Sometimes swelling makes things worse. It doesn't matter what causes the problem. Pursed-lip breathing is the answer. It can get you out of trouble when you are short of breath. It can prevent episodes of shortness of breath.

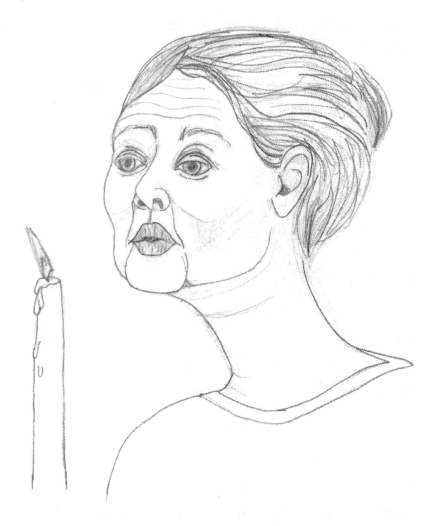

So sit back and relax in your favorite chair. Take in a nice deep breath, and then let it flow back out through lips that look like you could be whistling or kissing. It doesn't matter how you get the air in, mouth or nose. It only matters that there is slight back pressure slowing the breath as it leaves your lungs.

Once you have been practicing for a few minutes, add Step 2.

Step 2—Slowed exhalation

What makes this step so easy is that you are probably already doing it. Just using pursed lips slows your exhalation, and if you pay attention, you will probably find you are already breathing out for about twice as long as you breathe in. You can test the theory by counting to yourself. Breathe in to the count of three and out to the count of six.

That's a good place to start. It is not important that your ratio be exact. Everyone is unique, and you should find the ratio that is right for you. The point is that it should be somewhere around 3:6. If your ratio is more like 3:3, you are probably not really relaxing enough and not getting the full benefit of the breathing technique. If your ratio is more like 3:24, then you are missing about three breaths in and you will feel it!

Still easy, isn't it?

I have found that it is a good idea to spend a few days practicing just this part of the basic breathing exercise before you add the third, more difficult step. A good time to practice is while you are watching TV or reading. If you connect practice with something that happens almost every day (reading the paper, maybe?), then eventually you don't even have to think about it. Practice will just come naturally when that activity occurs.

If you never move on to the third step, or if you find the third step too difficult, you still have a skill that will be useful every day. How is that? Well, slow pursed-lip breathing will help you walk farther without shortness of breath. Slow pursed-lip breathing will help you move a chair or pick up a grandchild more easily. Slow pursed-lip breathing may even get you up a flight of stairs that you never thought you would go up again. Slow pursed-lip breathing is what you go to when an emotional upset sends you into just the opposite: rapid, shallow breathing.

Maybe most important, once you master slow pursed-lip breathing, you never have to be afraid again. You will always know that you have a tool to get you out of shortness of breath. You can stop the cycle of shortness of breath that leads to panic, which leads to more shortness of breath, which leads to more panic, and so on.

We will go into all of these in more depth later. For now, I just want you to be motivated!

Chapter 3

When Good Lungs Go Bad

Something to Think About

As demonstrated by the first chapter, the lungs are fairly simple and easy to understand when they are healthy and doing their job. They are more complicated in disease, of course, but one thing remains simple. The lungs have only three ways to demonstrate that they are in trouble. No matter what is wrong with the lungs, what part of the system is affected, or how it is affected, there are only three possible symptoms.

Those three symptoms are 1) shortness of breath, 2) mucus production and coughing, and 3) low blood-oxygen level. You may be thinking 1 and 3 sound like the same thing, but they are not. They often go hand in hand, but not always. You can feel very short of breath from working hard to breathe, but a test of oxygen level shows that you are succeeding with all that hard work. The flip side is that some people get used to a low oxygen level and don't experience it as shortness of breath.

Things get complicated when we start talking about what problems can cause those symptoms. The most common problems fall under the label COPD.

COPD stands for Chronic Obstructive Pulmonary Disease.

C stands for "chronic," which means the problem is going to stick around for a long time. It is not curable and not fatal (at least not for a long time), so it is chronic.

O stands for "obstructive," which will be explained next.

P stands for "pulmonary," which means related to the lungs. (They tried calling it COLD for a while, but that just sounds silly.)

D means "disease," and most people know that means illness.

COPD. Most of it is easy to understand. It is just the "O" that needs explaining. It stands for "obstructive" and that means there is a problem or obstruction to breathing *out.* Most lung diseases are obstructive.

The opposite of obstructive is "restrictive," and that means the problem is breathing in. Now, you may be thinking that you must have the restrictive type because your problem is breathing in. But remember, the brain never screams, "Breathe out! Breathe out!" It always demands another breath in, even if the reason you can't get a breath in is that you haven't cleared enough space by breathing out.

In obstructive lung diseases, which are by far more common, it is hard to breathe in because the lungs are still partly filled with the last breath. On top of that, the fresh air that does get in has to mix with the stale air left behind, so the oxygen level is lower.

This is very important information, because you can learn to override the brain's message and work on getting the last breath out BEFORE you take the next breath in. That is a huge part of symptom control. Very often an episode of shortness of breath, which can be so frightening, can be resolved quickly just by simple pursed-lip breathing, the technique you learned in the last chapter.

There are three common obstructive lung diseases and one less common one. The first three are emphysema, chronic bronchitis, and asthma. The fourth is called bronchiectasis. Simply put, emphysema is damage to the air sacs. Chronic bronchitis is damage to the bronchial tubes. Asthma is an abnormal reaction in the bronchial tubes. Bronchiectasis is just like chronic bronchitis, but with a different cause and worse symptoms.

Now we'll go into them in more depth.

EMPHYSEMA

To understand emphysema, we have to go back to learn more about the air sacs themselves. They are tiny air-filled sacs at the end of the bronchial tubes where the real work of the lungs takes place. Each one is surrounded by tiny blood vessels that pick up the oxygen out of the air and drop off the carbon dioxide. In normal, healthy lungs, there are 300 million of them.

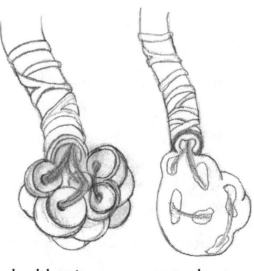

healthy air sacs   emphysema

That number is three times what you need to breathe completely comfortably. We all lose air sacs every day, because we are all getting older every day. But with normal wear and tear on the lungs you will never lose enough of them to be symptomatic. Unfortunately, smoking is not normal wear and tear on the lungs.

Smoking, and sometimes inhaling secondhand smoke, speeds the aging process in the lungs. Air sacs are destroyed more quickly, and you can lose two-thirds of them and have symptoms of shortness of breath.

The shortness of breath is caused by two things that are going on in your lungs when you lose air sacs. One is that there is not enough surface area left for gas exchange. By surface area I mean where air sacs meet blood vessels and oxygen crosses.

That sounds like a pretty big problem, but it is not really the biggest problem. The biggest problem is that the air sacs are used to help hold the bronchial tubes open, and with fewer air sacs the bronchial tubes lose support.

To understand this, you have to picture the inside of the lungs as more complex than just tubes leading to balls, the "bunch of grapes" picture we often have in our minds. A truer picture of what the lungs look like, if you were looking through a microscope, is a sponge or a slice of bread. The two major structures, the air sacs and the bronchial tubes, are all intermingled and wrapped around each other. They are so tiny and fragile that they need the surrounding tissue (each other) to remain open.

When the bronchial tubes don't have the support they need to stay open, they can collapse. But they don't collapse when you are breathing in. The rush of air itself keeps them open. They collapse when you are breathing out because, although you still have air moving that might keep them open, you have the chest wall coming down on them as well. Some bronchial tubes, not all, will collapse before you have finished breathing out.

In emphysema, the collapsing bronchial tubes cause the obstruction to exhalation and hence the "O" in COPD.

The air left behind is called trapped air. Obviously, if the lungs are already partially filled by trapped air, it is hard to get the next breath in. And the fresh air is diluted by stale air left behind.

Interestingly, the primary symptom of emphysema, shortness of breath, is caused far more by the increased work of breathing than it is by the lower oxygen level. We know this because it is easy to test for oxygen level. A simple clip on the finger can read what percentage of your red blood cells are carrying oxygen. During most episodes of shortness of breath, your oxygen level stays the same or close to the same. That means you may be working hard to breathe, but you are successful at it. The discomfort is caused by the *work* of breathing.

This should be reassuring, because it means you don't have to be so frightened when you are short of breath. Most of the time you are just uncomfortable, but not in any real danger. Plus, once you get practiced at pursed-lip breathing, you can relieve the discomfort and get some control of the situation back again.

I should mention at this point that heredity does play a role in who gets emphysema and who doesn't. We all know people who have smoked their whole lives and not gotten sick. They were fortunate enough to have been born with tough lungs, lungs that can take a lot of abuse. It is hard to know when you are a teenager and take up smoking whether you are going to be one of those people with tough lungs or not. You can guess at it by looking at your family history. But only time and living will tell.

There is one form of emphysema that is strictly hereditary. It is rare, but we suspect it when a nonsmoker gets emphysema or when someone very young does. It is called alpha-1 antitrypsin deficiency emphysema, because it is the lack of that enzyme that allows air sacs to be lost more quickly than the aging process can lose them and more quickly than smoking can destroy them.

If you suspect you have that form of emphysema, talk to your doctor about it. There is a test for it. It is an expensive test and one that insurance may not pay for unless there is a strong possibility that you have the disease. In other words, if you have smoked for any length of time, that is a far more likely cause for your condition than a hereditary defect, and your insurance company may not see the need to look further.

CHRONIC BRONCHITIS

While emphysema is damage to the air sacs, chronic bronchitis is damage to the bronchial tubes.

Remember that the bronchial tubes have that very special inner lining that catches dirt, pollution, and germs that are in the air we breathe and prevents them from making it down to the air sacs where they can cause pneumonia. When that lining is damaged, it doesn't do as good a job of protecting the air sacs.

In chronic bronchitis, the mucus-producing cells produce too much. On top of that, there are areas where the cilia, those fine hairlike projections that move the mucus up and out of the lungs, can be destroyed. Sometimes the cilia are still there, but they don't move like they are supposed to. As a matter of fact, cilia are paralyzed by cigarette smoke, so if you are still smoking, chronic bronchitis symptoms will be worse.

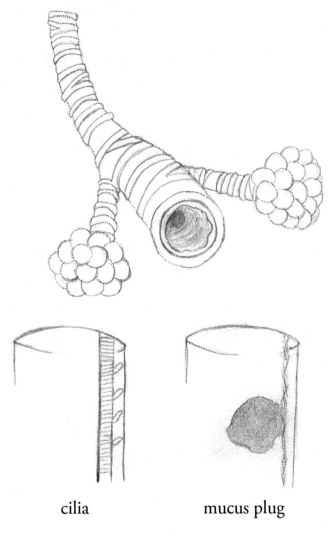

cilia   mucus plug

So if you picture that there is too much mucus in your lungs, and it is no longer creating a nice blanket lining the bronchial tubes, but clumping up, you can see the problem. The mucus plugs obstruct breathing. They obstruct breathing out, not breathing in, because the bronchial tubes are smaller on exhalation than they are on inhalation. Air can get around the plug on its way into the lungs. It is blocked on the way out. Hence, the "O" in COPD.

So the mucus plugs in the airways cause the same symptom of shortness of breath that collapsing airways cause in emphysema. Same symptoms, different cause, same breathing technique to resolve: PURSED-LIP BREATHING.

However, the mucus problem in chronic bronchitis causes an added problem: infection. The mucus blanket is no longer so effective at moving germs out of the lungs. Areas of infection occur in the bronchial tubes where germs (viruses and bacteria) have been allowed to stay in one place and set up shop. Infection causes even more production of mucus and even more destroyed cilia.

The good news is that there are ways to fight the mucus problem.

Think of it this way. The blobs of mucus in your lungs have three choices. They can stay in one place and obstruct breathing. They can drop down into the air sacs and cause pneumonia. Or you can cough them out. The best of the three, obviously, is coughing them out.

We can make coughing easier and more effective with bronchial hygiene techniques you will learn in a later chapter, but a hint for now is to drink more fluids. Thin mucus is easy to cough out. Dry little plugs are not.

So now you see that chronic bronchitis has more symptoms than emphysema. Although they both are characterized by shortness of breath, chronic bronchitis also has coughing and infection. Many people have both chronic bronchitis and emphysema. That makes sense because they both have the same cause most of the time, and that is cigarette smoke.

ASTHMA

Asthma is the third disease that falls under the heading COPD.

I always say that asthma is exactly like emphysema and chronic bronchitis AND it is completely different. It is just like the other two diseases because they have the same symptoms: shortness of breath and mucus problems. Much of the treatment is the same too. It is the cause of the symptoms that is completely different.

Unlike the other two diseases, in asthma, the structures of the lungs are not damaged. There are still plenty of air sacs and the bronchial lining is intact. The problem in asthma is an abnormal *reaction* in the bronchial tubes. That reaction is a swelling that decreases the inner diameter of the bronchial tubes. And as we already know, the bronchial tubes are already slightly smaller when breathing out than they are when breathing in, so the air may get in all right. It will have trouble getting out, some of it squeaking by the tight airways, hence the wheeze that is the hallmark of asthma, and hence the "O" in COPD.

So during an asthma attack, much like an episode of shortness of breath in the other two conditions, the brain may be screaming, "Breathe in! Breathe in!" but the real problem is that there is no room for the next breath when the last breath is still trapped in its place.

You have to override the brain and concentrate on breathing out first, then in.

Another thing that happens in asthma is that the irritated airways can produce extra mucus. So cough can be a symptom along with shortness of breath.

In theory, between asthma attacks the lungs are completely normal. The reason I add "in theory" is that for some people there is very little in-between time. It is just bad times and not-so-bad times. This is especially true for older people with asthma and asthma that accompanies the other two conditions.

That's right. It is not uncommon to have all three of the major obstructive lung diseases. The first two often happen together because they are both usually caused by cigarette smoke. Asthma may come along next because the thing that is irritating the lungs into the abnormal swelling is the fact that you have the other two conditions.

That may not be bad news!

It sounds like bad news when the doctor who has already told you that you have emphysema and chronic bronchitis tells you that he suspects asthma, but what it really means is that your symptoms may be more treatable than you think. Swelling can be treated with medication. There is no medication that grows back air sacs or brings cilia back to life.

But it is not so simple to say the asthmatic reaction, the swelling, is caused by the irritation of the other two diseases and leave it at that. There are many irritants that can cause the reaction.

Sometimes the cause and effect is obvious. Some asthmatics are allergic to things like cat dander or dust or pollen. Other times it is a mystery what causes the bad times and the not-so-bad times.

Unlike emphysema and chronic bronchitis, asthma isn't caused by cigarette smoke. Asthmatic airways (often called reactive airways) may react badly to cigarette smoke and usually do. But it doesn't cause asthma in otherwise healthy lungs.

We don't know what causes asthma. We don't know why I can live with eight cats but someone else would walk into my house and immediately start wheezing. Asthma tends to run in families. But it is not caused by families any more than it is caused by cigarette smoke.

I say that because there was a time when asthma was thought to be an emotional illness, caused by poor parenting. The wheeze was called the "maternal cry," meaning that the asthmatic child was crying out for more attention from his mother.

None of that bears any resemblance to what we know of asthma today. It is a very real physical condition, with very real physical causes. We just don't know what those causes are.

BRONCHIECTASIS

I said there were three major diseases and one minor under the heading of COPD. Bronchiectasis is the minor one, not because it is any easier to live with but because it is far less common.

Bronchiectasis is much like chronic bronchitis. The problem is in the lining of the airways, where mucus is overproduced and the mechanism for moving it up and out of the lungs is impaired. The difference is that in bronchiectasis there are actually pouches that hang off the bronchial tubes that harbor the infection. It is harder to get the mucus out and to treat the infection because it is hiding.

Bronchiectasis is not caused by smoking. It may be hereditary or it may be caused by trauma to the lungs. Children who inhale a foreign object may have damage to the bronchial lining left behind that gives them bronchiectasis. Sometimes, much like asthma, the roots bronchiectasis are a mystery.

Restrictive Lung Disease

Restrictive and obstructive are opposites when it comes to lung disease. The restrictive lung diseases DO NOT fall under the heading COPD. They may still have shortness of breath and coughing as the primary symptoms, but the causes are different.

In restrictive lung disease, the problem *really is* getting the air into the lungs. When the brain screams, "Breathe in! Breathe in!" it is right on target. The reason it is not easy to breathe in is that the lung tissue has become scarred or thickened. It has lost its stretchiness, so it won't easily let the air in.

One way to picture the difference between the two conditions is to picture two balloons. A lung with obstructive disease resembles a balloon that has been blown up for a long time and when the air is let out, it never regains its old shape and size. That balloon is easy to get air into but harder to get air out of.

A lung with restrictive disease is like a brand new balloon, one that is so tight that it hurts your cheeks to blow it up. A perfect balloon, just like a perfect lung, is one that air moves easily into and out of.

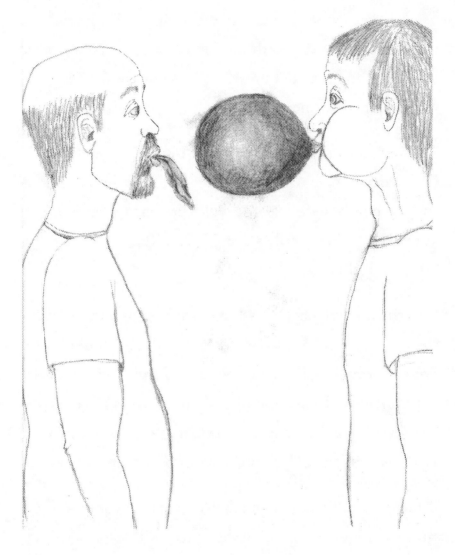

Most occupational lung diseases, like black lung from coal mining, are restrictive. Thanks to the Occupational Safety and Health Administration, we don't see much of that any more. The 9/11 first responders who have developed breathing problems probably have restrictive lung disease. Occasionally, the lungs react badly to a medication and scar tissue is left behind that causes a restrictive condition. Sometimes we don't know what causes the condition, and it may be called idiopathic interstitial fibrosis or pulmonary fibrosis. The word "idiopathic" means we don't know the cause.

There are two reasons to talk about restrictive lung diseases. One is that people with them may have picked up this book and are now wondering if it will help when they have just learned they don't really have COPD. The short answer is yes. It will still help.

I have had many people with restrictive lung diseases in my classes over the years. I wondered myself if they would benefit from information that is geared toward a different problem, but they have. I have found that the breathing techniques help, even though it is hard to explain why. It may just be the aspect of relaxing and thinking about breathing that helps.

If there is a mucus and cough aspect to the condition, the same techniques for clearing the mucus will help.

So I would suggest continuing to read.

The other reason I talk about restrictive versus obstructive is that it is easy to add a restrictive component to our breathing.

A simple thing like tight clothes can make breathing harder because they add a "restrictive component." If you already have lung trouble, that is the last thing you want to do.

There are other things that add a restrictive component. Pain that worsens with a deep breath is a restrictive component. That is why someone with COPD should have their pain well managed if they go into the hospital for surgery, particularly surgery anywhere on the trunk.

Excess weight adds a restrictive component and should be avoided. If only that was as easily done as said! Exercise will be covered in a later chapter, as will nutrition, but for now, try not to soothe yourself with ice cream in front of the TV too often.

If I was faced with a new diagnosis of an incurable disease, that would be my inclination. But later I would regret it. So will you. That being said, if your weight problem is that you have too little of it, feel free to soothe yourself with ice cream in front of the TV—as long as you also do your breathing exercises in front of the TV.

Chapter 4

Step 3—Breathing with the Diaphragm

Something to Do

You might read the title "Breathing with the Diaphragm" and think that can't be too hard. Isn't that how you breathe naturally? It may not be. Remember when we went over the muscles of respiration and said the diaphragm was the major muscle and there were extra help or accessory muscles in your neck, your shoulders, your upper back, and between the ribs? You can picture those extra-help muscles working if you picture a runner at the end of a marathon leaning on his knees and catching his breath with what looks like every muscle in his upper body.

Having those extra-help muscles is a real gift. Everyone uses them from time to time. When you have lung disease, you need them and use them more than ever. With obstructive lung diseases, where there is trapped air slowly accumulating over the years, that trapped air lowers the diaphragm, but doesn't let it relax back into as high a position in the chest as it used to relax into. The trapped air displaces it, so the distance it can move up and down with every breath becomes less and less as the years go by, sometimes long before you even know you have lung trouble.

The less the diaphragm moves, the more the accessory muscles have to help. Sometimes, as the disease progresses, the accessory muscles do the majority of the work of breathing and the diaphragm barely moves at all.

One way to know when you are relying on your accessory muscles is your posture. When they are doing the work, you may find yourself leaning a lot. You may be leaning forward with your hands on your thighs when you sit. You may find countertops or furniture to lean on when you stand. You do that to give your accessory muscles support while they work. It is called the tripod position.

Again, thank goodness the accessory muscles are there. But there are problems when they do the majority of the work:

1) Pain—These muscles were never meant to work this hard. They can ache and spasm in protest.

2) They are not available to do their real job. The shoulder and upper chest muscles are supposed to help you use your arms. Every time you carry a bag of groceries

into the house or wash your hair in the shower, you need those muscles. If they are helping you breathe, they can't help you with anything else.

3) You no longer have anywhere to go when you need extra help. You don't have extra-help muscles if they are already doing the work of routine breathing.

You can learn to bring the diaphragm back into the picture, but how much so varies from person to person. Some people feel they have switched back to using the diaphragm as the primary muscle of breathing with enough work on it. Other feel they have made the diaphragm the extra-help muscle, but at least they know how to call it back into service when they need it. Most people get some benefit from working on adding Step 3 to the basic breathing exercise. But it does take work.

Here is my experience after teaching people with COPD. A week after I show them how to exercise their diaphragm, they will say that it is really hard and doesn't seem to be helping. Two weeks after I teach them, they will say it is getting easier but doesn't seem particularly useful. Three weeks after I teach them, they will walk into class and say, "You are not going to believe what I did yesterday."

Remember, the diaphragm is a muscle, so it is not going to get stronger overnight.

After all that preparation for how important—and how difficult—this exercise is, here is how to do it:

The best position for this exercise is reclined. Lie back in your recliner, or put some pillows at the end of the couch to lie back on. Get comfortable and put your hands on your tummy. Do some pursed-lip breathing first to relax.

While you are pursed-lip breathing, look at what your tummy is doing. Does it move up and down with every breath? Is it lifting your hands? Does it lift while you inhale or while you exhale?

If your tummy lifts your hands when you breathe in, that is exactly what it is supposed to do. If you are using your diaphragm, it lowers with each breath in and the abdominal contents (or tummy) get out of the way by pooching out.

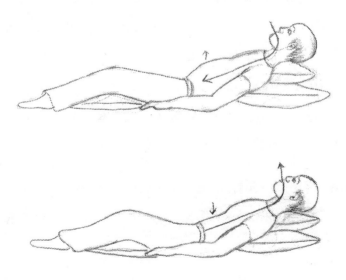

If your body is already doing it right, that is great news.

If, like most people with lung disease, your tummy lifts while you exhale or doesn't lift at all, you've got work to do. The work is to coordinate tummy lifting with inhaling. Picture the air filling up your lungs, pushing down on the diaphragm at the bottom of your lungs, and your tummy lifting to make room for those air-filled lungs.

If you are having trouble with it, just do two or three breaths, and then put it aside for now. Next time you try you may get to four or five before it gets too difficult. But that is progress.

The reason your tummy wants to lift as you breathe out is that you are using your accessory muscles to breathe in instead of your diaphragm. They make room for the air by lifting your shoulders and your upper ribs. If you try it right now, as an experiment, lifting your shoulders and upper chest as you take a breath in, you will see that your tummy automatically sinks in. When you let that breath back out again, your tummy will rise back to the old position.

For many people with lung disease, this has become the primary way to breathe. This exercise is meant to reverse that, to put you back where you were five or ten years ago, breathing with your diaphragm.

So lie back and practice several times a day, at the beginning. Get as many correct breaths in and out as you can. Remember, air in, tummy out. Put your hands, or maybe a tissue box, on your tummy so you can watch it lift up with every breath in and slip back down with every breath out.

When it gets too hard, or if you get lightheaded or feel it is making you more short of breath, put it aside for a while. It will get easier as the muscle gets stronger. You will be able to do more in a row with time. In a few weeks, if you keep with it, you will begin to believe me that there is a benefit to this.

If lightheadedness is what stops you, or if your fingers begin to tingle, you are working too hard, moving too much air. Just slow it down or don't breathe quite so deeply, and see if that helps.

If you get short of breath doing this exercise, you might need to speed it up. If someone could count your breaths while you exercise, know that the normal rate of breathing is twelve times a minute. If you are breathing eight or nine times a minute, that may be why you are short of breath.

For many patients, this part of the exercise eventually gets as easy as pursed-lip breathing and the slowed exhalation. For others, it is work, but worth it. Every now and then I run into a patient who just can't pull the diaphragm back into the habit of breathing. If you find yourself in that last category, don't worry too much. You still have pursed-lip breathing. And like I said at the beginning of this chapter, pursed-lip breathing is the most important thing I can teach you.

Chapter 5

Complications of COPD

Something to Think About

The hardest question to answer in a class of patients is "Will this disease get worse as the years go by?" It is a hard question because it is a hard answer. Yes. COPD is a progressive disease. Some of the downhill progress is just the aging process. We all get worse every day after a certain age, right?

But some of the "getting worse" is because of complications. A bout of pneumonia will drop your level of functioning, especially if it is caught late and gets very severe. And that is why it is so vital that we talk about complications. They can often be avoided or minimized if caught early. That can slow the progress of this progressive disease significantly.

There are three common complications of COPD: pneumonia, heart failure, and exacerbation.

PNEUMONIA

Pneumonia is infection in the air sacs of the lung. With infection comes mucus. Mucus is a good thing when it forms a nice blanket and carries germs out of the lungs. It is not so good when it accumulates as plugs in the bronchial tubes. It is life threatening when it lands in the air sacs and blocks oxygen from crossing into the bloodstream.

Another thing that makes pneumonia so serious is that the infection crosses easily into the bloodstream, creating a sickness that affects the whole body. High fever, extreme fatigue, and shortness of breath are nothing you want to mess with if you don't have to.

Sometimes pneumonia just springs up out of nowhere. You go to bed feeling well one night and wake up sick in the morning. When that happens, there was no opportunity to detect it early and possibly no way to prevent it. The pneumonia shot might have prevented it. Although it does not protect against all types of pneumonia, it does prevent the most common type.

But often pneumonia starts with an infection somewhere else in the respiratory tract and is carried down into the air sacs by your breath. So the first step in avoiding pneumonia is to avoid colds, the flu, sore throats, and sinus infections.

An immunization against the flu will decrease your chances of getting sick and is highly recommended, just like the pneumonia shot.

Beyond that, you could just avoid all human contact and then be assured of not catching anything. For most, that would be a dreadful existence, so the key is avoiding *unnecessary* human contact, and then deciding what contact is necessary.

For example, if you go to church on Sunday, that is a lot of exposure to colds. Only you know what going to church is worth to you and whether the exposure is necessary or unnecessary. A compromise might be to go to a service that is less well attended.

Family is a source of infection, especially young children, who sometimes seem to have a constant runny nose. A compromise to avoiding the people we love is letting them know in advance that they should stay away when they have a fresh cold. Viruses like the ones that cause colds are most contagious in the first few days, so that grandbaby with the constant runny nose is probably not contagious any more.

However, there are always get-togethers that are too important to miss, even if someone does have a fresh cold. You wouldn't want to stay home alone on Christmas Day, for example. Loneliness isn't good for you either.

So when people with germs are unavoidable, keep this in mind: cold germs are spread by hand more than they are spread by air. That doesn't mean it's a good idea to kiss the baby with the fresh cold. It is not *impossible* to get a cold from someone who sneezes in your face! Just keep your hands away from your face if you have had hand-to-hand contact or have picked up things that others have touched. Wash your hands frequently.

You will probably still catch some colds. If someone in your own household is sick, no amount of avoidance will keep the germs from you. Plus, colds are also contagious on the day before the symptoms appear. So a realistic goal is to catch fewer colds—and to pick up the signs as early as possible.

The first sign may be an increase in symptoms you already have, such as coughing.

If you are more tired than usual, more short of breath, or coughing more, it might be the first sign of an upper respiratory infection. But it might not be too. If you are not sure, try two things. Look at what you cough up. And take your temperature.

Yellow, green, or blood-streaked mucus might signal that you are coming down with something, especially if your mucus is usually white or clear. A low-grade fever, anything less than 101, is another early sign. (A fever over 101 isn't early any more. Call your doctor.)

What are you going to do if you decide you are getting sick? Four things:

1) Rest.

2) Drink more fluids; double your usual amount, if you can do it.

3) Talk to your doctor about antibiotics. It's an individual decision, not one-size-fits-all.

4) Clean that mucus out of your lungs.

Everything on that list, except rest, needs further discussion. Let's start with drinking more fluids. The amount that is recommended seems like a lot to me, eight glasses a day during healthy times and sixteen when you are getting sick or think you are. My advice is to do the best you can and make it easier by following a couple of simple tricks.

Unless you are a person who enjoys drinking water all day (some do), keep a variety of things you like around the house.

Have a selection of interesting teas and/or juices. And keep something next to you to sip as the day goes by. That might increase your chances of making it to that sixteen-glass-a-day goal.

Notice that I said teas and juices, not beer and soda! That doesn't mean other drinks are offlimits. It just means you need to be aware of a couple of things. Alcohol doesn't loosen mucus. It dries it up. If you do have a beer or a glass of wine, it doesn't count in your sixteen-glass total. Too much alcohol can also depress your drive to breathe and cough, thus increasing your chance of ending up with pneumonia.

Caffeinated drinks should be limited, because you want to sleep too, don't you? And sixteen sodas a day could put you on a sugar high. Milk can cause increased mucus production for some people, so moderation should be the watchword on those types of drinks.

As for antibiotics, that is between you and your doctor. There was a time when they were used liberally to prevent pneumonia in COPD patients. Doctors would give patients a course of antibiotics to keep at home and decide for themselves when to use them. But that was before the advent of super-infections. We know now that overuse of antibiotics has its own set of problems.

The key for you is to report accurately to your doctor what is going on with you. What is your temperature? What color is your mucus? How long has it been that way? Your doctor might decide not to use antibiotics right now but ask you to call again the next day with an update on your symptoms. He is not blowing you off. He is doing the right thing, waiting to be sure antibiotics are really needed before he prescribes them.

And the last thing you need to remember is to take the whole course of antibiotics any time they are prescribed. If you stop early, perhaps thinking that you feel better already and can save the rest of the pills for the next lung infection, you are risking starting a super-infection in your own lungs! You may have killed the weakest bacteria with the antibiotics and left the strongest behind, giving them a chance to reproduce and start the next infection. Do that a few times and you are growing yourself a powerful germ.

Bronchial hygiene means just what it sounds like it means— keeping your lungs clean. Drinking lots of fluids is the first step in keeping mucus loose enough to cough out, but it is not enough. In the past, bronchial hygiene has been a complicated ritual involving hanging off the bed to get gravity on your side, having a relative pound on your chest to knock the mucus loose.

But luckily, some genius invented a gadget called an airway agitator that allows you to vibrate the mucus loose from the inside out just by blowing into it. The first version was called a Flutter valve. A more recent one is called the Acapella. Both are simple, cheap, and very effective.

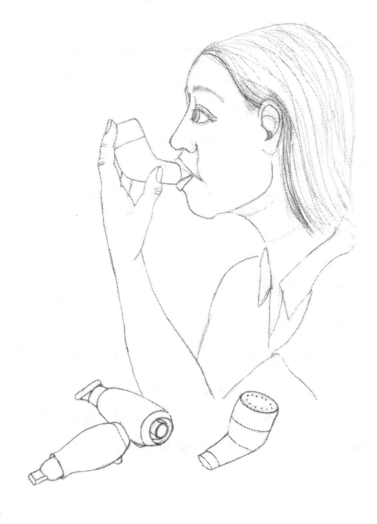

So here is what a bronchial hygiene break might look like:

1) You are already drinking lots of fluids, but right now a hot drink will help loosen things in your chest.

2) Use your inhaled breathing medicine (Albuterol or Combivent) to open your airways wide.

3) Pick up your airway agitator and blow into it—three easy breaths first, then three hard, deep breaths.

4) Wait a few moments and make yourself cough.

Using this technique, you will get out mucus that might otherwise stay in your lungs and cause pneumonia. Repeat the bronchial hygiene break several times a day, maybe every time your inhaled bronchodilator is due, every four to six hours.

If you have a mucus problem even on a good day, I highly recommend making a habit of taking a bronchial hygiene break every day, preventively. Morning is the ideal time of day, to get up anything that may have accumulated in your lungs overnight. Bedtime is the worst time of day, as it almost guarantees you will be up coughing all night.

HEART DISEASE DUE TO LUNG DISEASE

The second complication of lung disease is a condition called cor pulmonale, or heart failure caused by lung disease. It happens when the lungs don't deliver enough oxygen.

There are several reasons why the lungs might not deliver like they used to. There is not enough surface area for the oxygen to cross into the bloodstream in emphysema. There may be mucus plugs in the way in chronic bronchitis. In any obstructive lung disease, there is trapped air diluting fresh air. In restrictive lung diseases, the oxygen may be having a hard time crossing thickened or scarred tissue.

No matter what the cause, low blood oxygen is a problem and it causes more problems.

Because every muscle, tissue, and organ in the body requires oxygen, all of them suffer when there is not enough. You might not think as clearly because your brain is affected. You might be weaker because you muscles are affected. You might not digest food as well because the stomach is affected.

All of these are unpleasant, but it is downright dangerous when the heart is affected by low blood oxygen. First, the heart speeds up to compensate for the problem. It's a trade-off of quantity for the lack of quality. Second, capillaries in the lungs constrict or get smaller as a result of low blood oxygen. That means the right side of the heart, the side that pumps blood to the lungs, has to work harder. So now we have the heart working harder and faster. How much can we ask of it!?

For some people a third problem is that the blood thickens when there is not enough oxygen. The bone marrow, where red blood cells are made, mistakenly thinks the problems is lack of red blood cells to carry the oxygen, so it makes more. So now we have the heart working faster and harder to push thicker blood through smaller spaces.

Eventually, we have just asked too much of the heart. We have created high pressure between the right side of the heart and the lungs. As long as the pressure stays in the segment of the cardiovascular system, there are no added symptoms. The problems arise when the pressure becomes too much and it starts backing up into other parts of the system.

I think of it like traffic on a busy highway system. If there is a breakdown, causing a lane to be out of use, the traffic will still flow freely most of the time. But when rush hour comes, every lane is needed and the resulting backup of traffic is like the pressure in that one segment of the cardiovascular system. Both backups are likely to get worse before they get better. In the big city, cars start getting off at an earlier exit to avoid the backup. In the body, the serum of the blood starts getting off at an earlier exit, anywhere it can. The feet are the most likely place because gravity puts them already at higher pressure. When the serum of the blood starts seeping into the tissues, you get swollen feet and ankles.

That is a problem when you are trying to get your shoes on, but it is also a warning of things to come.

A little bit of fluid escaping the system is not going to relieve pressure for long. The backup is going to continue until the whole cardiovascular system is under high pressure. This means the pressure is felt all the way back to the lungs from both directions now and some of the fluid is going to try to escape across the membrane that oxygen is supposed to cross. This means there will be fluid in the lungs blocking gas exchange.

The problem has just become life threatening.

If it gets this far and you are rushed to the hospital, they will begin helping in the ambulance by giving you oxygen. When you get to the hospital a dose of Lasix, a diuretic, will get the fluid out of your lungs. But the whole episode will have been so traumatic for your body that you will probably have to stay in the hospital a few days and will come out functioning at a lower level than when you went in.

The solution? Detect the problem at the earliest possible moment.

The good news is that most doctors' offices have a simple gadget that clips on your finger to read your blood-oxygen level. If you go to the doctor regularly, any downward trend will be noted.

If you don't get it checked, or if your blood-oxygen level goes down quickly for some reason (maybe a lung infection), then your swollen ankles will give you a warning of worse things to come. The trick is to heed the warning so you don't have to get to the ambulance and emergency room stage.

The bad news is that the way to avoid this problem altogether, the early treatment that goes along with the early detection, is supplemental oxygen.

For many people with lung disease, the green tank and the plastic tubing under the nose is a deal breaker. I don't know how many patients have said to me that when that time comes, they would just as soon die.

I tell them it is their choice to make as long as it is an educated choice. As long as they understand that death is the likely alternative to using home oxygen and that they may be cutting many happy and productive years off their life. As long as they have a true picture of what they are putting their heart through by walking around with a low oxygen level.

I can count the ones who continued to refuse home oxygen on one hand. When push comes to shove, most of us will do what it takes to stay alive.

These days it is not uncommon to see someone grocery shopping with a tank of oxygen in the cart, or enjoying a picnic with family, plastic hose draping behind them. There was a time when oxygen signaled that death was near, but not anymore. In lung disease, oxygen is not a death sentence, but a reprieve from one.

Because oxygen is a medication, I will go into it in more depth in the chapter on medications.

EXACERBATION

The American Heritage Medical Dictionary defines "exacerbation" as "an increase in the severity of a disease or any of its signs or symptoms." An exacerbation of COPD means a worsening of the symptoms, primarily shortness of breath, with no other explanation.

I list it as the third complication because it happens so often in COPD that you should be prepared for it. Basically, it goes like this: You get worse. You go to the doctor or the hospital. They look for and don't find signs of infection or heart failure. They may put you on a higher dose of your breathing meds for a while. Then you get better.

Maybe someday we will know what triggers these spells or what is going on in the lungs that makes you feel worse. But we do not know that now. The key is to take it easy for a while and know it will pass.

Chapter 6

Improving Your Exercise Tolerance

Something to Do

By learning how to steer clear of the complications of lung disease, you can slow down its progression. But by exercising regularly, you can actually turn back time with regard to your lung disease. That doesn't mean that you can grow back air sacs or heal damaged bronchial tubes. But you can improve your body's ability to cope with the disease you have.

In the years that I have taught people to live with lung disease, I have seen for myself what a difference exercise and or regular activity can make. I have often had people sitting next to each other in class who were living proof. I have had a woman with mild lung disease who can barely walk in to class from the car sitting next to a man who has severe lung disease but still works a construction job.

The difference is that the man working construction has kept the rest of his body in top condition just by going to work every day. The woman, who had retired from a desk job, had let her muscles deteriorate even as her lungs did.

It is easy to see why she would retire to the TV set. Shortness of breath is a pretty frightening experience, so avoiding it is a natural response. The problem is that the limits you set for yourself become the limit of your possibilities. You can't sit in front of the TV and let your family take care of you, then suddenly decide to go out and do your own Christmas shopping. Inactivity, not disease, will have turned you into an invalid.

The trick is to stop being afraid of shortness of breath.

Ideally, by the time you are ready to start building your exercise tolerance, you have been practicing pursed-lip breathing for a while. You have seen for yourself that you can regain control of your breathing fairly quickly if you just focus on emptying your lungs before you try to fill them again. Just a moment or two of pursed-lip breathing can get you back in control.

Pursed-lip breathing as you exercise can prevent shortness of breath or at least delay it until you have accomplished all you want to accomplish on a particular day.

Exercise can mean anything from walking around the house to going to a gym and using the exercise equipment. For myself, I prefer to keep it simple. For many patients, there is no choice but to keep it simple. If you are already debilitated and hoping to build up again, getting to the gym alone can use up all the energy you have. Many a patient has started their exercise routine at walking from the bed to the chair. You have to start where you are.

The goal is to walk a little farther every day or every chance you get until you find the peak of your abilities. If you are walking from the bed to the chair, have someone move the chair farther every few days. With pursed-lip breathing, you will get there every time. If you are starting with walking to the end of your driveway and back, add a few yards every day. The worst that can happen is that you will have to stand in one place for a moment and pursed-lip breathe yourself back into control, but you will make it.

If you are lucky enough to be starting with long walks, it may actually be time to invest in a treadmill or join a gym. You may be surprised how much of a motivator a gym can be, just because of the camaraderie. Or find a pulmonary rehabilitation program. There you will get the education you need, as well as regular exercise monitored by a professional. Pulmonary rehab is not for everyone because of the time and money commitment, but it may be right for you.

Motivation is hard to maintain when it comes to exercise. A good trick for staying motivated is to keep a record of how you are doing. A simple legal pad with a few columns can help you see how far you have come at a glance. You could label five columns with the date, type of exercise, distance, results, and goal for tomorrow. If you finish today and feel you could have done more, make that your goal for tomorrow. If you feel like you pushed yourself to the limit, plateau for a while. Make your plan for tomorrow the same as what it was today. It may be a week before you think you can add more.

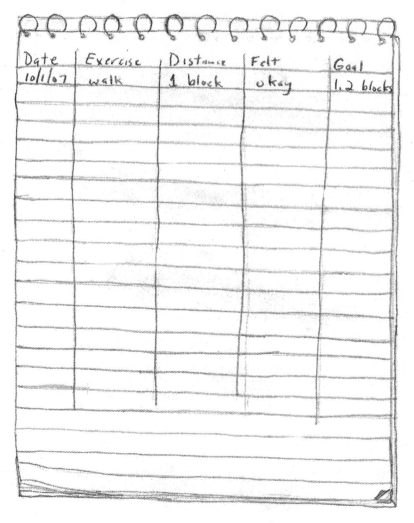

Date	Exercise	Distance	Felt	Goal
10/1/07	walk	1 block	okay	1.2 blocks

But when you get frustrated, you only need to look at the records you keep to see how far you have come.

If you get sick in the middle of your attempt to build your exercise tolerance, it is okay to take a break while you get your health back. Just start up again as soon as you can. If you start up again and see you have lost ground, looking at your old record can remind you that you can build again. You did it once. You can do it again.

I emphasize walking as an exercise because I am a firm believer that it is more important to build your leg muscles than any other muscle except your diaphragm. Your legs determine your level of mobility, and mobility determines quality of life.

I think most would agree that being bed bound is a very poor quality of life compared with being able to walk around your own house. Being able to get around only your own house is a poorer quality of life than being able to get out and do your own errands. Legs determine your abilities to take care of yourself. Legs determine your level of independence and therefore your quality of life.

Walking isn't the only way to build your leg muscles. It is just the most obvious. An exercise bike is a good alternative.

A treadmill is an alternative to walking around the neighborhood. You decide which method works for you, but try to do a little more all the time, with the help of pursed-lip breathing. Keep a record, not only to stay motivated, but to dazzle your doctor!

Chapter 7

Medications and Gadgets

Something to Think About

At first glance "medications" seems like a huge topic. There are so many medications you could be on. Most people with lung disease have a kitchen counter lined with pills and inhalers. But I can make this simple for you.

First of all, you may be on medications for other problems, and I am not going to try to tackle all of them. You should know what pills are for what problem, but for our purposes, scoot everything to one side that is for blood pressure or arthritis or anything other than lung disease. We will just focus on what remains.

To simplify things further, you won't be taking any medications to cure your disease. There is no cure at this moment. All of your medications are about controlling symptoms, and you will recall that there are only three possible symptoms of COPD.

So all of your medications are prescribed to deal with one of three things: breathing problems, mucus problems, or heart problems caused by low blood oxygen. We will talk about each category separately.

MEDICATIONS FOR BREATHING PROBLEMS

There are two types of medication to treat shortness of breath. Bronchodilators firm up your bronchial tubes so they don't collapse so easily, and steroids prevent or treat swelling in the bronchial tubes.

Most bronchodilators are inhaled medications. Every now and then a pill comes out that claims to be a bronchodilator, but they haven't stayed on the market for long, so either they don't work well or they cause too many side effects.

Aminophylline is a pill that was used to dilate the bronchial tubes. It has gone in and out of fashion over the years but is currently out of use. The problem with it was that it could cause heart rhythm disturbances and you had to have a blood test done regularly to make sure you weren't getting too high a dose. When it was the best we had, it was considered worth the risk and inconvenience. There are so many new and better and less risky meds out there now, I doubt we will see it again. But I could be wrong about that, so I mention it here.

The most commonly used bronchodilator is albuterol. It is inhaled, either from a metered dose inhaler or a nebulizer. It acts quickly and lasts four to six hours.

Another similar drug is called Atrovent. Atrovent takes longer to kick in, fifteen to twenty minutes, but it actually does a better job of holding the tubes open. Interestingly, when given the choice of the two, most people chose albuterol because speed was the most important factor.

Fortunately, some brilliant drug company came up with the idea of putting the two together in the same inhaler so you could get the best of both worlds. That medication is called Combivent.

Another improvement on albuterol and Atrovent dreamed up by the drug companies was to make them longer acting. Albuterol was made into the longer-acting Serevent. At first Serevent was very popular. You had to take it only twice a day, so you didn't have to suffer from shortness of breath every time your medication started to wear off four to six times a day. You didn't have to wake up short of breath in the middle of the night because your medication had worn off.

The problem with the longer-acting Serevent was that it contained three times the medication in each puff from the inhaler and people who took it for relief from an acute episode of shortness of breath could overdose very quickly. An overdose can cause your heart to beat very fast. That might not be a serious problem for most people. Our hearts speed up with activity, with emotion, with all kinds of triggers in the course of the day. But if you also have heart trouble, and it speeds up too much, it could be serious enough to require an ER visit.

Serevent is still around and you may be on it. If you are, you should still have Albuterol as a rescue inhaler. It can also speed up your heart, as it is essentially the same medicine, but it would take three times as many puffs. Plus it works quickly so you may not be tempted to take too many puffs.

Atrovent has also been developed into a long-acting version, called Spiriva. It is a much more recent addition to the arsenal of medications for shortness of breath, and so far, all the news is good. There are few to no side effects. And you have to take it only once a day. The interesting and really wonderful thing about this medication is that you take it every twenty-four hours, but it works for thirty-two hours. You experience no symptoms of having taken too much during those hours when the two doses overlap. And there is no breakthrough shortness of breath when the medication is wearing off. It doesn't have a chance to wear off.

The only negative thing I can say about Spiriva is that it doesn't work for everyone. It either works wonders or it doesn't work at all. From my experience with patients, it usually works wonders.

That might be the end of the story of bronchodilators. Spiriva once a day and albuterol as a rescue inhaler seems to be the obvious and best combination. Inhaled steroids complicate matters. Drug companies have combined them with bronchodilators in medications you hear advertised on TV, such as Advair. Not everyone needs an inhaled steroid as well as a bronchodilator.

If your doctor thinks you would benefit from an inhaled steroid, you should talk about your options. Convenience is worth considering. Before long-acting inhaled medications and combination medications, you could have found yourself on three different inhalers, one three times a day and two four times a day, each requiring two puffs separated by a minute. Life revolved around the clock and a bag of inhalers.

Things are easier now, but you still have to decide whether the convenience of one inhaler is worth giving up the long-acting Spiriva.

But we shouldn't go any further before we talk about steroids in general. Steroids are quite a bit different from bronchodilators. They are not only for lungs and they are not only inhaled. Steroids are used in pill form and also in IV form if you are in the hospital. They are used to treat anything where swelling or inflammation are causing symptoms.

Steroids were considered miracle drugs when they were first developed. Not only could they tame the swelling that caused asthma attacks, but they relieved the pain of swollen arthritic joints. They caused mood swings in some people, but often the swing was to the positive side, so who cares, right?!

But like most miracles, time told a different story. Prednisone, the most commonly used steroid pill, had some unexpected long-term side effects, including diabetes, muscle wasting, and bleeding ulcers. Plus, once on it for a few years it was nearly impossible to stop it, because the body had adjusted to it and would not readjust easily.

So prednisone, although still used for acute breathing problems, is used more carefully than ever before. If you are having an exacerbation, your doctor may prescribe a prednisone "taper." That means he will start it at a high dose, forty to sixty milligrams, and have you decrease the dose gradually over the next weeks. If you have to stay on prednisone, your doctor will make sure you are on the lowest possible dose.

Inhaled steroids solved a lot of the problems prednisone caused. The idea behind them was that they worked by coating the inside of your lungs and bringing down the swelling from the outside in. The steroid itself did not have to get into your bloodstream to work.

Inhaled steroids actually were a miracle for some people, particularly people who were able to use them instead of prednisone. But it turned out that a small amount still leaked into the bloodstream. And there can be some local side effects, such as a yeast infection in the mouth.

Therefore it is important to take inhaled steroids properly. Cough and clear the lungs of excess mucus beforehand. Rinse your mouth well afterward.

You might notice that things keep changing when it comes to medications. What is considered the best today may be second best tomorrow or even completely out of use. That is not true of other things in this book. I have been teaching breathing exercises since the mid-seventies. They helped then, and they still help today.

Medications, especially breathing medications, keep changing. There is a way, however, to find the latest information. Ask your doctor about something called the GOLD standard for care of the COPD patient. That isn't "Gold" as in gold jewelry, but GOLD, standing for Global Initiative for Chronic Obstructive Lung Disease. Those are standards of care agreed upon by the medical arm of the American Lung Association and the World Health Organization. If your doctor does not know what that is, call your local chapter of the American Lung Association and ask for a copy to be sent to you. Take it to your doctor. With it, and information from your breathing tests and your history of complications, he can decide whether you should be on inhaled steroids or what bronchodilator would be best for you.

You may not find the right medication or combination of medications immediately. You may react differently than expected to a medication just because you are a unique individual. Your reaction, and your sense that things are getting better or are not, is more important than any GOLD standards. Don't be too surprised if you have to work with your doctor for a while to find the medications that are right for you.

MEDICATIONS FOR SECRETION PROBLEMS

Let's move on to problems created by mucus. You may remember that the mucus blanket lining the bronchial tubes is a great thing when it works properly. It defends the more fragile air sacs from infection. When irritation from cigarette smoke or anything else disrupts the mucus blanket, you end up with a cough if you are lucky, an infection if you are not lucky.

Coughing is a symptom, because it is annoying, but it is still the best alternative for excess mucus. If you take a cough medicine, you want it to be an expectorant, not a suppressant.

Expectorants are mostly over-the-counter medications. You don't need a prescription for Robitussin or anything else that is right there on the drugstore shelf. They work to loosen mucus so it is easier to cough up. A good fluid intake does the same. You can try them and see if they work for you. If they do work, it probably won't be a dramatic change. Only you can decide if it is worth the expense.

Cough suppressants are usually a bad idea. You need to cough to get the mucus out. Not only does it block the air movement in your lungs, but it carries infection, which can cause bronchitis or pneumonia.

Most over-the-counter cough suppressants don't work well enough to lead to serious problems. They are too mild. There are stronger cough suppressants available by prescription.

Although it is usually a bad idea to suppress your cough, there is one exception to that rule. Sometimes you get a dry cough that just won't go away and won't let you sleep. It seems like the sleeplessness is making you rundown and having a negative effect on your health in general. You and your doctor may agree that a good night's sleep is a high priority. He may give you a prescription for something strong—the "big guns."

The one I am thinking of is called Tussinex and I personally can attest to the fact that it works. Just remember, when you wake up in the morning after the medication has given you a good night's sleep, you may have accumulated mucus in your lungs that needs to come up. Take a hot shower (if that helps you loosen mucus), drink a hot drink, and take your rescue inhaler. Use your airway agitator. And cough, cough, cough.

Now, let's say all your efforts to avoid infection haven't worked this time. You are running a low-grade fever and the stuff you are coughing up is green. The medication you'll be taking is an antibiotic.

There a so many different antibiotics, I won't try to list them here. Your doctor will probably prescribe a "broad spectrum" antibiotic. That means it kills all the common bacteria, the ones you are most likely to get in your lungs. If you take it for three or more days and don't feel any better, or especially if you feel worse, call your doctor. He may want to send a sample of your mucus to the lab to find the exact right antibiotic for you.

I've said it before, but it is important enough to repeat: when you are prescribed an antibiotic, take the whole course of it. If you stop early, you may leave behind the strongest bacteria so they can reproduce and make your next lung infection even worse. If you do that a few times, you can end up with an infection that can be treated only with antibiotics that are wildly expensive and have terrible side effects.

If you want to stop the antibiotic because you think it is making you sicker, maybe adding nausea to your list of symptoms, call your doctor and ask for a switch to a new antibiotic.

There are herbal remedies that claim to prevent or treat colds. Echinacea is said to boost your immune system and is recommended when you feel a cold coming on. There are no studies that prove it helps, but there is also no information that it is dangerous. Clear it with your doctor, and give it a try.

Zinc is another over-the-counter remedy that comes in many forms, but I prefer the lozenges. The claim is that it shortens the duration of a cold. I take zinc when I get a cold and recommend it to all my friends. Again, make sure your doctor knows what you are taking, even if it is over-the-counter.

MEDICATIONS FOR HEART DISEASE CAUSED BY LUNG DISEASE

Only two medications are on this list, and the first is oxygen. Many people don't think of oxygen as a medication. There was a time when it was not considered one.

Forty years ago, when I was a nurse's aide, saying a patient was "on oxygen" was code for "near death." And the patient was probably under a plastic tent with 100 percent oxygen blasting into it. We thought of oxygen as something that made dying more comfortable back then, though it probably didn't.

We know now that the body requires a specific amount of oxygen. Too much can create as many problems as too little.

If your lungs aren't delivering enough oxygen to the bloodstream, the strain on your heart can be life threatening. It is important that you add enough oxygen, usually one to three liters per minute by a nasal cannula, to take the strain off your heart. As we talked about in an earlier chapter, it can add years to your life.

If oxygen could be taken in pill form, there would probably be no resistance to it. But there is no such pill, and it is a difficult hurdle for many folks to jump, to accept the fact that they may need to be tethered to an oxygen tank, possibly for the rest of their lives.

I cannot emphasize enough that without the oxygen tank, "the rest of your life" is probably less than five years. With it, no limits apply. The advent of home oxygen took COPD from a "terminal" illness to a chronic one.

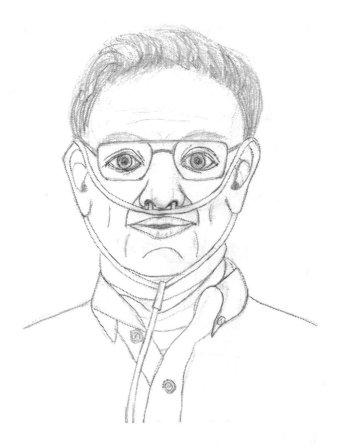

Your doctor will prescribe the amount of oxygen you use, just like any other medication. He will tell you how many hours a day to use it and what liter flow to use. He determines this based on your "oxygen saturation," the percent of red blood cells that are carrying oxygen. That is the number provided by that little clip they put on your finger every time you go near a medical professional. He will also look at your symptoms to make that call.

Studies show that very few patients use the oxygen as much as ordered. Many people make a mental compromise: "Okay, I will use it, but only when I am at home." Again, it is always your choice what to do with your own body. But when you are out and active, you may need it even more. It may not extend your life expectancy as much if you don't use it all the time prescribed.

Some people use it more than prescribed, thinking erroneously that it will do even more good that way. Some people turn up the liter flow when they use it to make up for the time they don't use it.

Using the oxygen at a higher liter flow than ordered is usually just a waste of oxygen. It may dry up your nasal passages more than needed. It may cause a headache if you really crank it up to five or six liters. But in rare cases, it can actually depress your drive to breathe, leading to a frantic trip to the ER.

And you can't store up oxygen for later use. Sorry.

In some cases, using home oxygen is temporary. For example, if you start using it while you have pneumonia and that clears up, a quick check with the clip on your finger may give you good news. If you live at high altitude and move to lower altitude, you may get the same good news.

But if you do need to stay on oxygen, there are alternatives to the green tank. That is actually something you can use when you go out. You will probably use something called an oxygen concentrator when you are at home. Ask the company that supplies your oxygen to tell you about liquid oxygen too. The portable version can be smaller and lighter than anything you have seen yet.

You might also take a diuretic if your heart has gotten involved in your health problems for any reason. Some people call it a water pill because it wrings the water out of you. It makes you pee more! The most common one is called Lasix.

Lasix works to take the load off your heart by decreasing the volume of circulating blood. It is like having less traffic on the highway when there is a lane closed. The system can still handle the decreased load.

If you are on a diuretic, you may have to have a blood test periodically to make sure your electrolytes are not being depleted.

And if you are on a diuretic, it may seem silly to also drink a lot of fluids to loosen your mucus. It may seem they are at crosspurposes. But the increased fluid intake manages to loosen the mucus *before* it is wrung out of the body by the diuretic.

I will be honest with you about one thing: you are going to spend a lot of time in the bathroom!

GADGETS

There are so many devices and gadgets out there to help with breathing, measure breathing, deliver medications, or bring up mucus, it can really get confusing. I will start by telling you what you don't need and can get rid of.

1) You don't need a peak flow meter unless you have pure asthma, without emphysema or chronic bronchitis. It is not accurate for anyone else.

2) You don't need an incentive spirometer unless you are in the hospital and just had surgery. It is meant to open up air sacs that have collapsed while under anesthesia. Your air sacs are too open, remember?

3) There are also gadgets out there that claim to exercise your breathing muscles. You will recall that the muscles of breathing are the diaphragm and the accessory muscles. It doesn't make sense to exercise the accessory muscles. They work hard enough already. And the diaphragm can be exercised just by doing the exercise

in Chapter 4. It may make sense to use this gadget if you have restrictive lung disease.

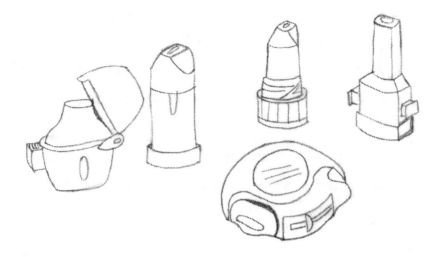

Here's what you might find useful:

1) An airway agitator like the Flutter valve or Acapella. Both gadgets that vibrate your lungs from the inside out are very worthwhile. Even if you don't usually have a mucus problem, a bad cold could cause one, and having that gadget handy could prevent pneumonia. Ask your doctor how to get one.

2) If you don't have something to vibrate your lungs from the inside out, you can always do it the old-fashioned way. Use a vibrator that you might have for a bad back and tuck it under your arm against your rib cage. If it

vibrates your vocal cords (your voice vibrates), then it is shaking your lungs up too and will help you get the mucus up.

3) If you use any medication that comes in a metered dose inhaler, a spacer will help you do a better job. It is a plastic cylinder that you attach to the mouthpiece of your inhaler. You will get the highest, most consistent dose of medicine into your lungs if you use it, and you don't even need great hand-eye coordination like you do if you use the inhaler alone.

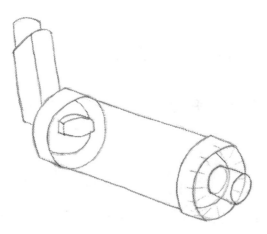

4) If you are on any of the newer inhaled medications, they might come in a different-looking package. Serevent and Advair come in a disc. The medication is pulled out by your breath, not pushed out by a propellant.

You don't need any gadget to go with them. You just have to read the instructions carefully. Spiriva is delivered by something called a HandiHaler. Some of the inhaled steroids come in their own unique delivery gadgets. Make sure you read the instructions for how to hold your head and how to hold the medicine canister while you take it. You can review the instructions with your pharmacist when you pick it up too.

5) Some people take their inhaled medications with the help of a nebulizer. That means you will drop a small amount of the medication into a plastic canister and an air compressor forces air through it, turning it into a mist. With a nebulizer, you just sit back, relax, and breathe. It takes a few minutes to get the whole dose in, but some feel they get more benefit from the meds that way. It's not as portable as an inhaler, and studies don't support that you get more medication from it. But most doctors support you if you say you need it, and so do I.

6) Oxygen saturation monitors have become cheaper over the years, so it is more common for patients to want to have one of their own. At first I thought this was a bad idea, that patients would become obsessed with

that one number and fearful of any slight dip. But for those who have purchased one, that hasn't happened. More often than not, the gadget has reassured them that they are okay. Plus if the number isn't reassuring, they know to get to the doctor or hospital. If you are interested in having one, call an oxygen supply company. The most recent information I have is that they cost about $400, and insurance does not help with that.

Chapter 8

Activities of Daily Living

Something to Do

Between shortness of breath and the fear of shortness of breath, it can be tough getting through the day with COPD. It should be easier once you get practiced at using pursed-lip breathing to get yourself out of trouble, but that doesn't solve all the problems you may encounter.

It doesn't help that it often doesn't make sense which activities are easy to do and which ones cause shortness of breath. And you can't find a solution until you determine the cause.

If you play detective, however, you may be able to figure out the cause. Consider these three possibilities:

1) You are inadvertently holding your breath.

2) You are using your arms, taking your accessory muscles away from helping you breathe.

3) You are inhaling something that irritates your airways.

Let's dig deeper into each possibility:

First, we hold our breath many times in the course of the day without even realizing we are doing it. You hold your breath, for example, when you lift something. You may be moving a kitchen chair from in front of the TV, or picking a baby up out of a crib. If you have normal, healthy lungs, it is fine to hold your breath. It strengthens your chest to, so to speak, close the trapdoor at the top of your lungs. And you do it for only a few seconds.

But when you have lung disease, that few seconds may be enough to throw off that fragile rhythm of breathing in and breathing out. Your lungs react as if you were holding your breath to swim the English Channel!

An alternative to holding your breath is slow, controlled pursed-lip breathing. For example, look at that chair you want to move, take a breath in, and then breathe out slowly against pursed lips while you lift and move the chair. When you set it down, take another breath in. See if it isn't easier.

There are other things you do in the course of the day that may involve breath holding. Lowering yourself into or lifting yourself out of the bathtub are a couple. Try pursed-lip breathing with that maneuver and see if it isn't easier.

As you bend over, whether to pull socks on or pick up the cat, breathe out through pursed lips. It is easy when you are pushing your diaphragm up with the maneuver anyway.

Pursed-lip breathing can help you go up a flight of stairs too. It may or may not be replacing breath holding. When I have asked patients how they usually go up stairs, most say, "As fast as I can to get it over with."

Here's a better idea. Stand at the bottom of the stairs and take a breath in. Exhale through pursed lips while you take a step (or two or three) up. When you need to breathe in again, stand still for the moment, then exhale through pursed lips again while you take a few more steps. Always stand still for the inhalation. Pursed-lip breathe for the steps up.

It will take longer, but at least you won't be standing at the top of the stairs gasping like it may be your last gasp!

Next, let's examine a question I get asked a lot by patients and their families. Why is it so hard to carry groceries in from the car? That is a perfect example of an activity that takes your accessory muscles away from breathing so they can help you use your arms. Even a short walk, even a light load of groceries, and suddenly you are gasping again. You don't realize it, but you are moving very little air when your accessory muscles of breathing have been given another job to do.

The solution to this one is to call on your diaphragm. This is when you will be glad you put the time in on the last step of the basic breathing exercise. Standing at the trunk of your car, do a few breaths with pursed lips. Remind your diaphragm to go out when you breathe in and in when you breathe out. Then pick up that sack of groceries and see how much easier it is!

Shampooing your hair is another activity that may be difficult if your accessory muscles have become your major muscles of breathing. If you get short of breath in the shower, try breathing with your diaphragm in that setting too.

If the shower is a particularly difficult time for you, it may be more than how you breathe. It may also be what you breathe, and that is the third issue we are going to discus here. Many soaps and lotions have perfumes that irritate your lungs. Try replacing them with scent- or perfume-free products.

If the steam makes you short of breath, you can cut down on it with better ventilation. Open the window or door a crack.

Use a slightly cooler water temperature. You might even get a handheld showerhead—the kind that is open and running only if you are squeezing it. In New Mexico they called that a Navy shower. It saves water *and* cuts down on humidity.

You might also consider getting rid of things that spray, like deodorant or bathroom cleaner. And if hairspray is one your life essentials, take a breath in before you spray, exhale while you spray, then leave the room as quickly as possible.

Next to showering, I think the hardest activity is putting fresh sheets on a bed. It combines using the arms with breath holding and even throws some dust into the air at the same time.

For years I have encouraged people to consider changing their sheets less often, but I have rarely convinced anyone. Another alternative might be letting someone else in the family assume that responsibility if it wears you out for the rest of the day.

Although it is great to learn how to get through the day with less shortness of breath, there is nothing wrong with avoiding an activity altogether if it is too much trouble and avoidable.

To me, energy conservation has always meant saving your strength for the things you enjoy or the things you really have to do. I would rather see you use the best part of the day to go for a nice walk than to change sheets. That way you can enjoy the weather and build up your exercise tolerance at the same time.

You can conserve energy in simple ways too, like leaving the pans you use a lot on the stove instead of in the cabinet or wearing slip-on shoes instead of ones that tie. It is not lazy to put yourself first sometimes. It is wise.

A patient told me once that the best advice she ever got was to buy a thick terry cloth robe to put on after she bathed. That way the robe did the work of drying her off and she didn't have to. I didn't give her that tip. She got it in a booklet the American Lung Association puts out called "Around the Clock with COPD." It was written by patients and has hundreds of little tips. They don't all work for everyone, but when you find the ones that work for you, they are not so little any more. I would advise everyone to call the Lung Association and get a copy.

Chapter 9

Emotional Aspects Of COPD

Something to Think About

I used to joke with my kids that you have to be brave only if you have a permanent illness. If you have something temporary, play it for all it's worth. That excused my neediness every time I got a bad cold.

The truth is, it is not easy keeping a stiff upper lip when faced with an illness that is not going to go away. It is a loss, just like losing a loved one or a job that you love. You may go through all the stages that grief involves, such as anger and depression. Everyone experiences things in their own unique way, so be kind to yourself while you get used to your diagnosis.

If and when you get to an acceptance of it, you will probably realize that most of us eventually have to live with chronic illness. Modern medicine has allowed us to live longer, but not necessarily in good health.

If smoker's guilt adds to your distress, remember what I said earlier. Most of our chronic illnesses will be the result of, or at least contributed to, by our own bad habits or carelessness. Smoking is not the only bad habit. Poor eating habits, drinking alcohol, even excessive time in the sun can come back to haunt us.

Like I said, be kind to yourself.

Sometimes family members make things harder when they could make things easier. They might be going through their own grieving process, if your diagnosis is new information. They might react negatively out of fear of losing you. They might also be angry if they tried to get you to quit smoking and you either didn't quit or didn't quit soon enough.

If it is possible to have a frank conversation about it, do it. Smoking is considered the hardest thing to quit. They say it is easier to quit alcohol or even heroin. Having run a smoking cessation clinic out of a pulmonologist's office, I can tell you that my success rate was never more than 60 percent. And these were people with lung disease who desperately wanted to quit. All you can do is your best. Let them know you did your best.

If there are other smokers in the family, you should all agree not to expose each other to secondhand smoke. That's not good for anyone, particularly children. Just going out on the porch to smoke will probably limit your number of cigarettes, so that might be a step in the right direction for everyone.

There are other things that are best talked about in advance, such as avoiding people with colds. If the first your family hears of it is when they are standing at your front door expecting to drop the grandkids off, there can be hard feelings.

It doesn't lead to any better feelings if you go ahead and take the grandkids, catch the little one's cold, and end up in the hospital with pneumonia.

One thing about lung disease that can affect family relationships is that you may not look sick. Family members may see you doing things you enjoy, like gardening, and think that means you can do anything and everything for yourself. It doesn't make sense that you can't carry a sack of groceries in the house but can do so many other things. It does make sense once they understand about using the accessory muscles to breathe.

Again, sit down and have a conversation about lung disease. Or hand them this book to read.

The flip side of not looking sick when you have lung disease is that during an episode of shortness of breath, you look more than sick. You look like you are going to die! Anyone who witnesses a bad episode may become overprotective, not allowing you to do anything for yourself. That may feel good for a while. And it is okay for a little while. But if your muscles go unused, they can become useless pretty quickly. It is easier to keep them in good shape than it is to restore them later.

Reassure your family that you can still do quite a bit for yourself. Show them, if the opportunity presents itself, that you can breathe your way out of shortness of breath. But you might also take them up on offers to do things that really are difficult for you. This might be an opportunity to get someone else to change the sheets on your bed.

Or, for example, if you have friends or family members (a teenage grandson, maybe) who keeps asking what they can do to help, ask them to come by on garbage day and bring yours out to the curb.

COPD may affect every relationship you have, but it also adds a new one to your life: the one with your doctor. And it is an important relationship. Choose wisely.

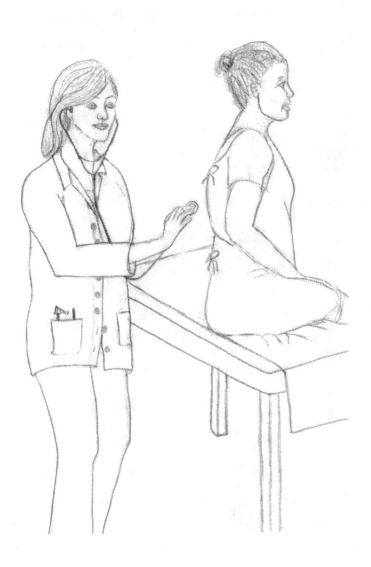

It is usually not necessary to go to a lung specialist, or pulmonologist. The general practitioner or internist or family doctor you already see may be just fine. If you stay with your generalist, though, don't be surprised if he isn't familiar with the GOLD standards or if you have to tell him about some new bronchodilator. They can't be experts on everything.

I would be concerned if any doctor responded negatively to you bringing him new information. I would be concerned if he doesn't like being questioned. Now, more than ever, you need to feel like a partner in your own care. You need someone who respects you as a partner, not someone who makes you feel like a bother or responds to your questions defensively.

You should be able to ask your doctor what your last breathing test showed, or why a chest x-ray is being ordered, and get a clear and honest answer.

That being said, there are limits to how much time you can ask of your doctor. There are always other patients in line behind you. You can't expect your doctor to give you an anatomy and physiology lecture every time you ask a question.

For example, let's say you ask about the results of a breathing test and he says, "Last year your test showed your breathing to be 60 percent of what it would be if you didn't have lung disease. This year you are down to 57 percent. That is about what I expected." That's a pretty good answer. If you go on to pummel him with questions about things like how many air sacs you have left and what he would have done if the test had been worse than expected, you may find a doctor easing toward the door.

There should be the same mutual respect when it comes to phone calls. Your call should be returned on the day you make it. Likely, it will not be the doctor himself who returns the call, but a staff member who has spoken to him about your problem.

Your part in making this interaction go well is to have all the information the doctor will need at your fingertips. What is your temperature? How long have your feet been swollen? If you are asking for something specific, like an appointment or antibiotics, say so. A lot of time can be wasted with the staff going to the doctor about your call when he is between patients. He then has them call you back for more information. They have to catch him between patients again. And on and on.

I am familiar with this scenario because I worked in a pulmonolgist's office for a while. Believe me, you cannot go to the doctor and say, "Mrs. Smith just called and she can't get out of her own way today." You just can't!

If you decide you are not happy with your doctor, you have every right to find a new one. However, you might consider talking to your doctor about your complaints before you make the final decision to move on. It could turn out to be just the wake-up call he needs. Maybe he doesn't know how he comes across and will decide to do better. Maybe he doesn't know your phone calls haven't been returned.

Changing doctors should not be taken lightly. I would hate to see you get sick when you are between doctors. Do some research on who you might prefer having as a doctor. Ask friends and family members if they can recommend someone they see. If there is a support group for people with COPD in your area, that would be a great place to get a lead on a good doctor.

And speaking of support groups . . . there is no better place to express your feelings about having COPD than with a group of people who have it too. You can vent your anger, cry your tears, and laugh at yourself in a group like this. If there isn't one in your area, consider starting one. All you need is a place, and hospitals have conference rooms that are perfect for it. Notices in the paper are usually free.

You would get the benefit of having a support group yourself, but it might also give you a sense of purpose to get this group together where everyone can help each other. Just a thought.

Chapter 10

Stopping The Anxiety Cycle

Something to Do

As you can tell, I have worked as a nurse for many years. Some of those years were in the ER. There is a scenario I have seen all too many times that bothers me: People with COPD come in by ambulance. A family member has called 911 because of a severe episode of shortness of breath. By the time the patient gets to the hospital, he is feeling much better. The family arrives shortly thereafter and reacts with anger to see that this episode "wasn't real."

People can begin to see you as manipulative, using your symptoms to punish. Or they see you as emotionally fragile, someone who can't handle the ups and downs of family life anymore.

They might tell you that you need to learn to "control your emotions." I am here to tell you it is not your emotions you need to control. You are not a robot. It is your breathing you need to control when you become emotional.

You see, there is a cycle that occurs when you get emotional. Strong emotion causes you to breathe faster. When you breathe faster, you trap more air than usual. That trapped air gives you a sense that you can't get air in, and that triggers a small panic response. That panic response makes you breathe faster and trap more air. Round and round you go. The cycle of anxiety causes shortness of breath causes anxiety.

The only difference between you and me is that I don't trap air when I breathe faster, so there is no cycle. My point is that your problem is a breathing problem, not an emotional problem.

And you solve it with a breathing technique: PURSED-LIP BREATHING. You can slow your breathing down, release that trapped air, and deal with the problem at hand. Just like you did before you got COPD.

Chapter 11

Medical tests and Lung Disease

Something to Think About

If you are going to be a partner with your doctor, it helps to speak the same language. That language includes the results of the many medical tests and exams you will have over the years. Below is a brief language lesson.

THE STETHOSCOPE

I can just about guarantee that every time you see your doctor, or any doctor for that matter, they will listen to your lungs with a stethoscope. It is standard procedure, even if you don't have lung disease. The stethoscope doesn't amplify the lung sounds, but brings them closer and blocks out all other sounds. It allows the doctor to hear the air move through your lungs and get an idea exactly what the air is moving through. Is he hearing a lot of air sacs, or just a few? Is he hearing extra sounds, like mucus in the airways?

I think of the analogy of a tree again, the airways being like the branches of a tree, dividing and dividing and dividing again until they get very small and numerous. Now we add leaves to that analogy. If you have a big oak tree outside your window, it sounds different when there are a lot of leaves than when there are very few. The sound is much louder when there are a lot of leaves, right? The breath sounds in your lungs are also louder when there are a lot of air sacs.

There is also a different sound when it rains on your tree, right? You might hear the doctor describe your lungs as sounding wet, or "junkie." That means there is a lot of mucus or that fluid is accumulating in the bases.

My analogy falls flat when we talk about the sound of pneumonia in your lungs. If the mucus has fallen to the air sacs, they will be "socked in," no air movement, silent, but just over the area where the pneumonia is.

Wheezing is another sound the doctor is listening for. Wheezing is the sound of air squeaking by a tiny passageway. That passageway may be tiny because of the swelling of asthma, or because of a mucus plug. If the wheezing is throughout the lungs, not just in one spot, it is more likely asthma. You might hear the doctor say your lungs sound "tight."

BREATHING TESTS

Breathing tests are used to diagnose COPD in the first place. A simple one called spirometry can be done in any doctor's office and should be used to screen for COPD. That is the test when the respiratory therapist has you take in a deep breath and breathe out as hard and fast and long as you can. They may make quite a show of getting to you exhale hard, jumping up and down shouting, "Keep going! Keep going!"

I've had patients tell me they thought the therapist was a little nutty, but that's how we are trained to do it, to get your absolute best effort.

Spirometry gives you two important numbers, forced vital capacity (FVC) and forced expiratory volume in one second (FEV1). The first one, the total amount of air you breathe out, is compared with your "predicted" result. Predicted varies with height and age and gender. What you want to know is what percentage of predicted you are.

FEV1 should be three-fourths of FVC. For example, if your total FVC is four liters, there should be three liters breathed out in the first second FEV1. In COPD, that number goes down first. The obstructed airways make exhaling slower, and this is where it shows up.

If your screening spirometry shows you have COPD, the doctor may order more complex breathing tests. He should also repeat the screening spirometry at least once a year and in between if he wants to see how a new medication is working.

As you can see, breathing tests are pretty important.

CHEST X-RAYS

COPD is detectable on a chest x-ray because the diaphragm, or lower border of the lungs, will be flatter than it should be. But this doesn't show up early. By the time COPD is obvious on your chest x-ray, you already know you have it.

Chest x-rays are used to pick up complications, not to diagnose COPD in the first place. Pneumonia shows up as a whited-out area on the black lung fields. It can be anywhere in the lungs. Heart failure shows up as a white fluffiness at the bottom of the lungs where gravity would have the fluid accumulating.

Your doctor might order a chest x-ray periodically to rule out lung cancer, because that disease has the same risk factors as COPD.

ARTERIAL BLOOD GASES

Most blood tests are drawn from the vein, somewhere between your hand and your elbow, most often in the crook of your elbow. Blood gases have to be drawn from an artery. Blood gases show the oxygen and carbon dioxide level in the blood after it leaves the lungs but before it gets to the tissue level, where gases are exchanged again.

They are drawn from the inside of your wrist or your elbow. I'll be honest and tell you that it usually hurts more than a usual blood test. You can ask for the area to be numbed first.

The invention of the oxygen saturation monitor, that clip they put in your finger that tells what percentage of your red blood cells have oxygen attached, has cut down dramatically on the number of blood gases that you will have done. You already know from that clip how well your lungs are doing at picking up oxygen. The extra information from the blood gas is your carbon dioxide level and your pH (acid/base balance).

The carbon dioxide level tells how hard you are working to breathe. If you are working hard, the number goes down because you are blowing off carbon dioxide. The pH tells if this is a new change or an old one. Carbon dioxide is the acid in acid/base balance. If your work of breathing is off the norm, the body will adjust by changing the base to match it. But the body doesn't adjust quickly. If you have had a recent change in your condition (maybe developed pneumonia), your pH will be off. If the carbon dioxide is off but the pH is not, it is a gradual or old change.

Bottom line: if your pH is off, we are more worried. A blood gas is often ordered if you come in to the ER with shortness of breath.

ELECTROCARDIOGRAM (EKG or ECG)

An EKG is a heart test, not a lung test, but we know the heart can be involved in lung disease, so your doctor will probably want to check it from time to time. You might also be experiencing chest pain from the work of breathing, and the doctor would want to see if it is just that and not a heart attack.

An EKG shows if there is damage to the heart by the configuration of those bumps you see. It also shows if your heart rhythm is regular, fast, or slow. Typically in COPD, it is a little less regular and a little faster than normal. This is not dangerous, but worth noting. It is always good to know your baseline, or what is normal for you now.

OTHER BLOOD TESTS

There are some basic blood tests that we all get any time we are sick, that you will also get when you are sick and sometimes when you are not.

For example, a CBC, or complete blood count, can tell if you are anemic, which means too few red blood cells, or polycythemic, which means too many. Remember that some people react to low oxygen by making more red blood cells.

A CBC also shows your white blood cell count. White blood cells fight infection, and the body makes more when there is an acute infection. If you show up at the doctor's office coughing up yellow mucus and he orders a CBC, a slightly higher white blood cell count might lead to the conclusion that you have bronchitis, but a dramatically higher count may look more like pneumonia.

Electrolytes are also checked frequently, especially if you are sick. If you take a diuretic, your potassium level can be low, which is not good for heart rhythm. It might tell the doctor that you need a potassium supplement.

Knowing the basics about tests that the doctor orders allows you to talk about results in more detail. You can ask, "What was my FEV1?" instead of "How was my test?" The answer can be more specific and you can keep a record if you want to. I think I would.

It also means you can request a particular test if you see a reason for it. For example, if you haven't had a chest x-ray in a long time and a friend has just received a diagnosis of lung cancer, you might ask the doctor to order one so you can be reassured.

I think understanding a little bit about tests that are ordered allows you to speak the same language as your doctor. And that is a good thing.

Chapter 12

Make Your Diaphragm Work Harder

Something to Do

By now you are using pursed-lip breathing for all kinds of things. You are conquering your fear of shortness of breath. You are walking a little bit each day, right?

Now might be a good time to see what happens when you do your breathing exercise with a book on your tummy. See if your diaphragm can lift weights. Don't start with *War and Peace*. Choose some lighter reading and work your way up!

Chapter 13

Nutrition and COPD

Something to Think About

It is important to make healthy food choices when you have COPD, but it is also important to make happy food choices. You have lost enough when you have a chronic illness without losing Cokes and potato chips and root beer floats. I don't want to be the one to tell you to stop feeding your bliss.

The good news is that you can ease your way to healthier eating. If you have just gotten a diagnosis of diabetes, you would have to change your ways immediately. Junk food would be considered life threatening. With COPD, improving your eating habits is not a matter of life and death but a matter of energy and comfort.

Breathing takes more energy when you have COPD. Fighting infection takes energy. All this walking you are going to do to improve your exercise tolerance takes energy. You get that energy from the foods you eat. At the same time, you may have less of an appetite when you have COPD. Your shrinking appetite may be caused by the fact that there is actually less room in your stomach for food. The lungs, with their trapped air, take up more space than they used to. They put the squeeze on your stomach when they do that.

If you have ever eaten a really big meal, like on Thanksgiving Day, then found yourself short of breath, it may be because your full stomach put the squeeze on your lungs this time.

The lesson here is twofold. Don't eat that really big meal and make yourself short of breath. That is lesson one. Eat frequent smaller meals. That is lesson two.

That might actually make it easier to slip into better eating habits. You could eat three really healthy small snacks/meals a day and still have room for the fun foods the other three times you eat. Then as time passes, you could make it four meals a day that are high in nutrient value and low in sugar and other filler. Later, as you get used to eating healthier, you could go to five good meals a day and one treat.

A simple way to know what the best foods are is to shop mostly along the edges of the grocery store. That is where you find the purest food, the meats, the vegetables, and the fruits. The more processed foods are in the middle of the store. Simply put, processing takes the nutrients out and leaves the shell with lots of flavor for us to get hooked on.

But you can get hooked on healthy food too. Let's take macaroni and cheese as an example. That boxed brand is sure tasty. But you can buy elbow macaroni made from vegetable pasta and grate cheddar cheese into it. It's no harder to make, and better for you.

I traded in ice cream for grapefruit slices, believe it or not. At first I loaded the grapefruit up with sugar, but I slowly stopped doing that. Now I crave grapefruit as much as I ever did ice cream. Yogurt is another good substitute if sweets are your downfall.

If salty foods are more important to you, try making a big salad at the salad bar but throwing in a few olives or dill pickles. Salsa can make anything tastier, even Brussels sprouts. A handful of salted nuts is better for you than a bag of potato chips. More protein means more energy.

If the doctor says you should limit your salt intake, look for no-salt spices to flavor things up. You can also use fewer olives on your salad as time goes by and less salsa. Ease yourself over to unsalted nuts.

Nothing has to happen overnight. And as you recognize that you have more energy, you might find yourself motivated to get even healthier in your food choices.

We don't want to make food preparation twice as hard by having twice as many meals. Make it easy on yourself whenever possible. My grapefruit slices come in a jar. Crackers with peanut butter make a good and simple snack/meal. Campbell's soups are easy and come in low-sodium varieties if you need them. You can slice zucchini into tomato soup. You can make egg drop soup out of chicken noodle soup just by dropping raw egg you have mixed into it. If you like to cook and have some favorite recipes, make a double batch and freeze small containers of it that you can microwave and eat later.

If you are overweight, everything you do takes more energy, so losing weight will make you feel better. Look for the lower-calorie varieties of the foods you love. There are ice creams with no added sugar. You could have that for your treat-yourself snack/meal. Another tip for losing weight is to be aware of portion size. Eating out of a bowl instead of a bag, say of potato chips, can give you a better visual of exactly how much you are eating. Reading food labels helps too. A friend of mine who is a cardiac nurse tells me you should look for saturated fats and never eat anything that has more than four grams of saturated fat per serving. She also says you should never eat in front of the TV. But I hesitate to give advice I myself couldn't follow, so I will just put it out there. We shouldn't eat in front of the TV.

If you are underweight, you don't have enough reserve if you get sick. You are the rare person who will get this advice: Eat your dessert before your vegetables. Eat in front of the TV. Finish a whole bag of chips. Make yourself a milk shake in the middle of the day. Drive through Wendy's and get a root beer float.

You lucky dog, you!

One more issue to think about is comfort. By that I mean abdominal comfort. Two things that will really take the joy out of eating are gas and constipation. A gassy, bloated abdomen can fight for space with your lungs just like a full belly does. Carbonated beverages cause gas, as do fried foods and beans. If you notice something else that causes gas for you, make note of it and try to avoid it.

Constipation is a real misery when you have breathing trouble. There is a lot of breath holding involved in straining in the bathroom, and you don't need that. If you are drinking lots of fluids, that may be enough, but more fiber in your diet will help too. Vegetables, fruit, and whole grains will keep things moving along.

Lastly, take a multivitamin. That doesn't replace good nutrition! It just enhances it.

Chapter 14

Things to Do in Bed with COPD

Something to Do

SEX

This is going to be a very short chapter! What I know about sex and COPD can be summed up in a joke I heard on a Brad Paisley album. (Yes, Brad Paisley has jokes on his albums.)

You know you are old when your wife says, "Honey, let's go upstairs and make love," and your answer is, "Darlin', I cannot do both."

Pace yourself!

Your sex life won't be spontaneous anymore, but it doesn't have to be over. You need to sit down with your partner and consider a few things. What time of day do you breathe best? What position is easiest for you? What really matters to both of you? The answers might surprise you.

Talk about what you will do if you get short of breath in the middle of the action. Use your inhaler? Change positions? Have a sip of wine? I had one patient tell me he and his wife used the start-stop technique. When he needed to rest, his wife rubbed his back for a moment. When he was ready, he picked up where he left off.

If all else fails, buy a vibrator. Tell yourself it's for bronchial hygiene, but keep it lying on the bedside table for any other use that might pop into your mind.

Keeping your sex life alive can make you realize that you want to stay alive and healthy as long as possible. Plus that orgasm at the end will give you a rush of adrenaline that works just like a bronchodilator.

Well, I guess I did know a little bit about sex and COPD!

SLEEP

Maybe it's all right with you if your sex life is over, and the bed is just for sleep now. That's okay too. But what if your sleep life seems to be over too?

For most people there are two kinds of sleep problems—falling asleep and staying asleep. For those of you with COPD there is a third possibility: you could sleep too well.

The easiest problem to solve is trouble falling asleep. It usually means you are taking your rescue inhaler too close to bedtime. Albuterol has the side effect of making you feel "wired," but it usually wears off. Try taking it an hour or more before you go to bed, or not at all, if you can get away with it. If coughing keeps you awake, try taking a bronchial hygiene break early in the evening. Don't do it right before bedtime. That will defeat your purpose and guarantee that you cough when you want to sleep.

The other two problems are harder to solve. If you have trouble staying asleep, you may have to accept it and plan around it. The reason you wake up may be that your breathing gets less effective as you get into a deeper stage of sleep and you have to wake up to get back in the right pattern of breathing. If you accept that you will be awake during the night, you can have a book at the bedside to pick up. Some people move to another part of the house, watch a little TV, and then spend the rest of the night sleeping in a recliner.

Sleeping too well is the other side of the same coin. If your body allows you to sleep through ineffective breathing, you may wake up feeling lousy. Again, plan around it. Have your inhaled medications at the bedside so you can use them before you even get out of bed. Do some good hard

Chapter 15

Review

If this were really a series of classes instead of a book, I would end with a review. I would ask the class, "What is the most important thing you learned about living with lung disease?"

I hope the answers would be something like this:

"PURSED-LIP BREATHING to control shortness of breath!"

"Avoid colds or catch them early so they don't turn into pneumonia."

"Use your oxygen the way your doctor tells you to."

"Always finish the course of antibiotics."

"Talk to the people in your life so they understand what you are going through."

"Keep active so you can stay independent."

"Live life to the fullest in spite of your disease."

"Just breathe."

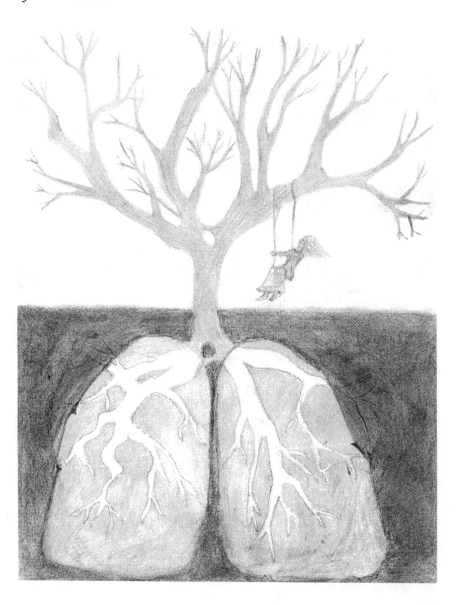

BIO

Mary Callahan is a registered nurse and a registry-eligible respiratory therapist living and working in Maine. She spent most of her 35 year nursing career focusing on patients with chronic lung disease, in hospital and out, teaching the Respiratory Disease Self-Care Classes, and making home visits.

She is the author of numerous magazine articles and newspaper pieces, as well as two other books. _Fighting for Tony_ is about raising a child with special needs. _Memoirs of a Babystealer_ is an exposé of the foster care system.

She is a mother of four, Tony, Renee, Michael and Bridget, as well as the grandmother of one extraordinary cover model, Melissa.